Simon Visits The Doctor

by Patty Lakin Koenigsberg
illustrated by Patricia Schories

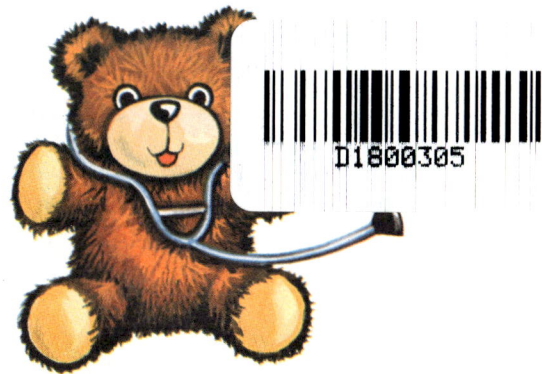

A GOLDEN BOOK • NEW YORK
Western Publishing Company, Inc.
Racine, Wisconsin 53404

Copyright © 1984 by Western Publishing Company, Inc. Illustrations copyright © 1984 by Patricia Schories. All rights reserved. Printed in the U.S.A. No part of this book may be reproduced or copied in any form without written permission from the publisher. GOLDEN®, GOLDEN & DESIGN®, A FIRST LITTLE GOLDEN BOOK®, and A GOLDEN BOOK® are trademarks of Western Publishing Company, Inc. Library of Congress Catalog Card Number: 83-83291 ISBN 0-307-10138-X ISBN 0-307-68156-4 (lib. bdg.)
FGHIJ

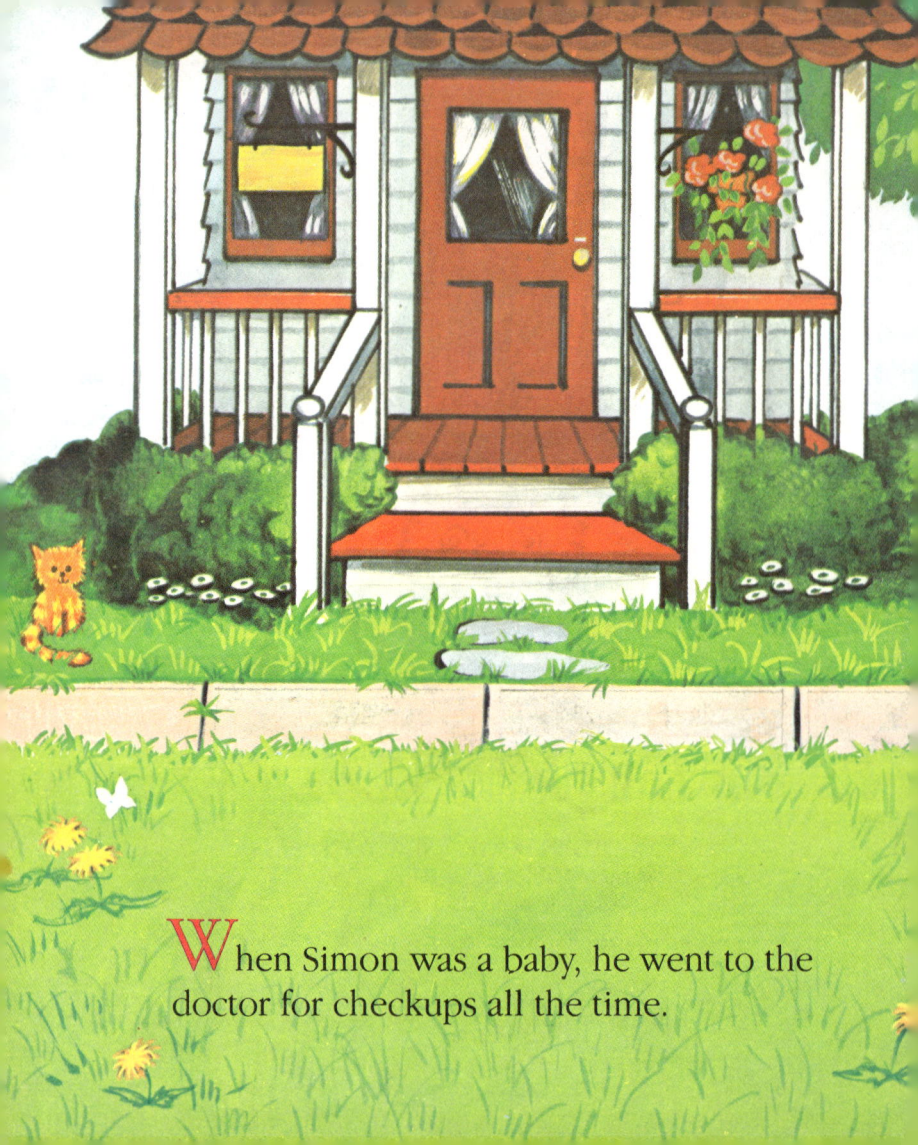

When Simon was a baby, he went to the doctor for checkups all the time.

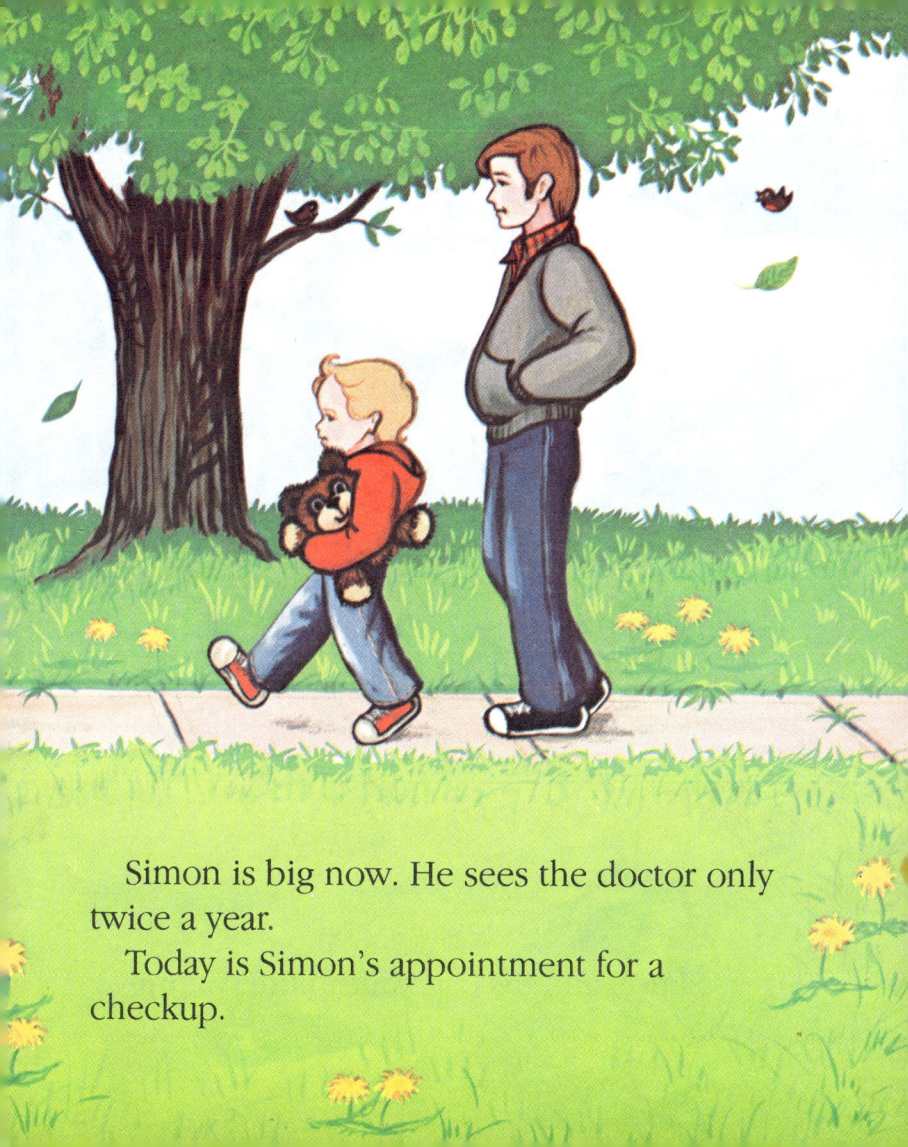

Simon is big now. He sees the doctor only twice a year.

Today is Simon's appointment for a checkup.

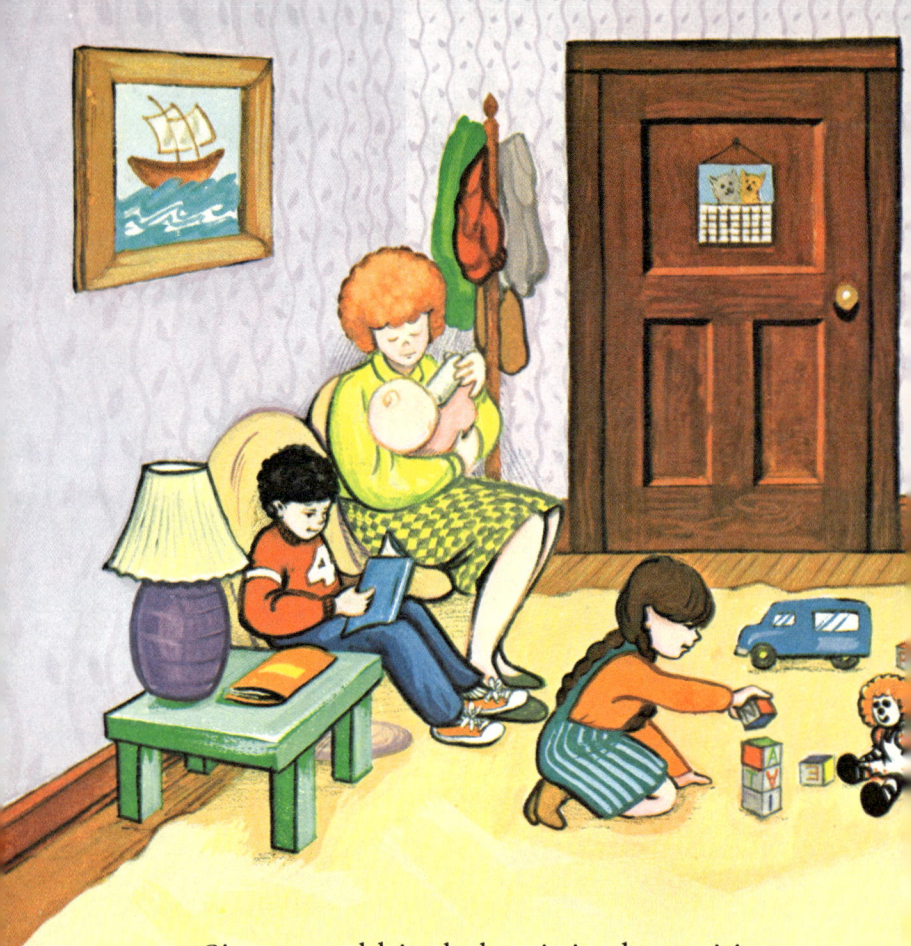

Simon and his dad wait in the waiting room.

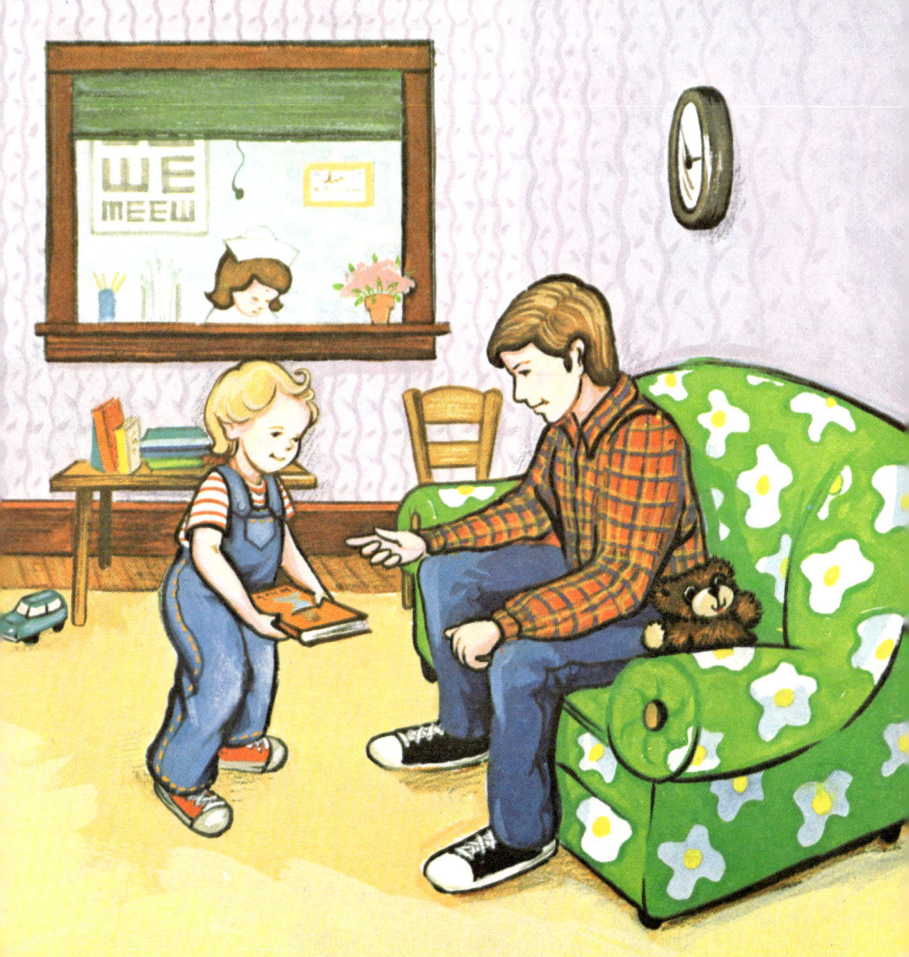

Simon asks his dad to read him a book.

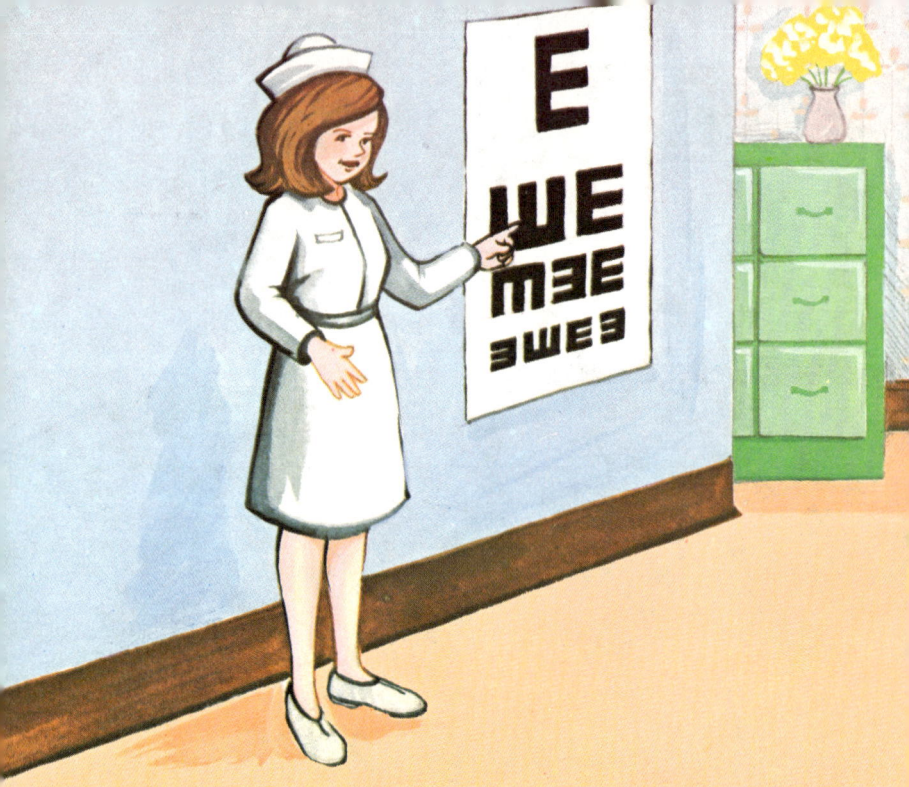

Mrs. Beach, the nurse, calls Simon into her office for an eye test.

She points to a chart on the wall. On it are E's that point different ways. Simon holds his fingers to show how the E's point.

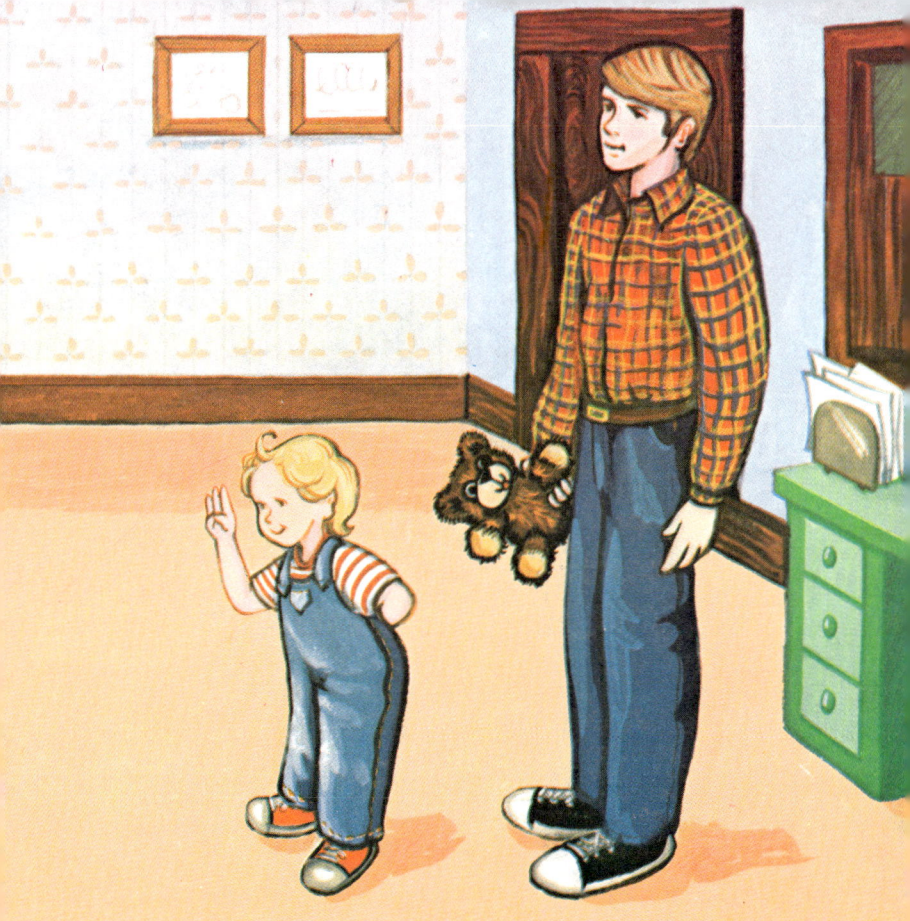

"Well done," says Mrs. Beach. "You have good eyesight."

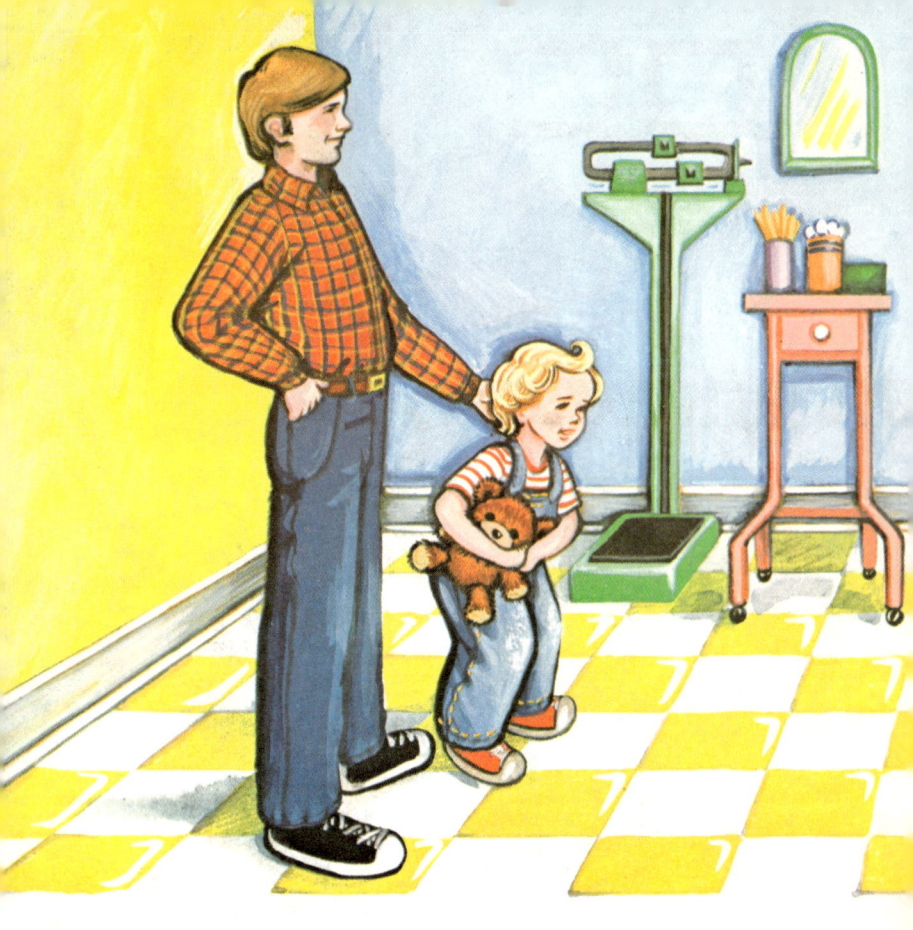

Then Simon and his dad go into
Dr. Smith's examining room.

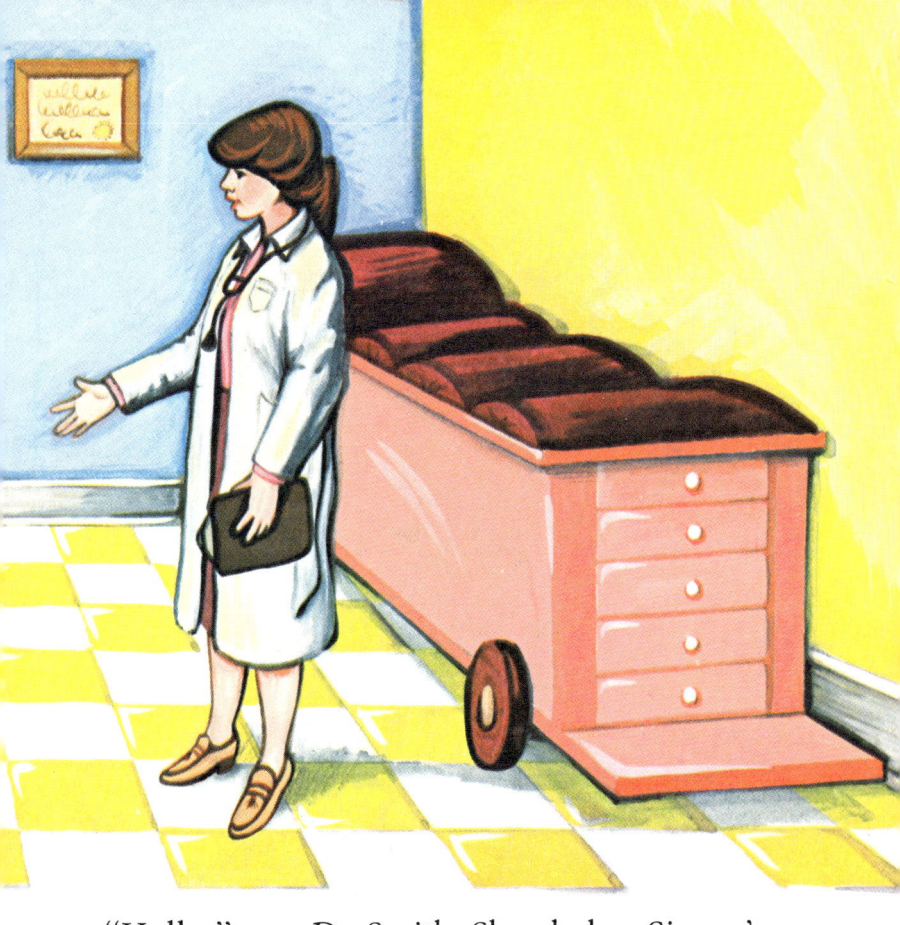

"Hello," says Dr. Smith. She shakes Simon's hand. "Hop out of your clothes, please, and let's see how much you have grown."

Simon takes off his shoes, socks, pants, and shirt and stands on the scale.

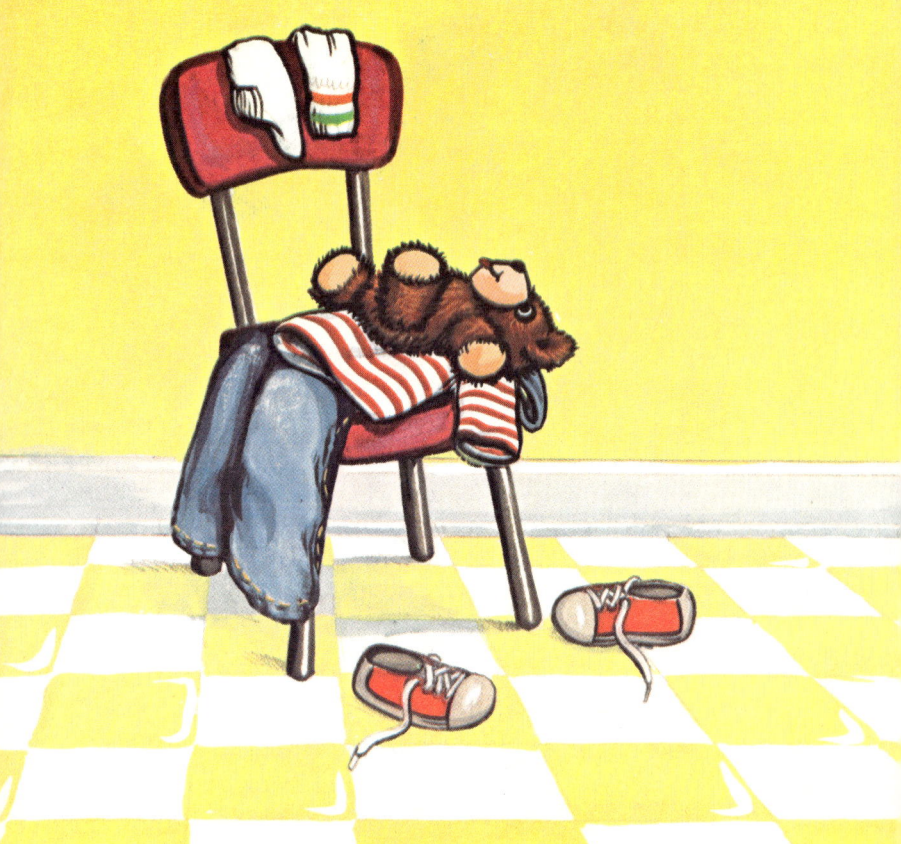

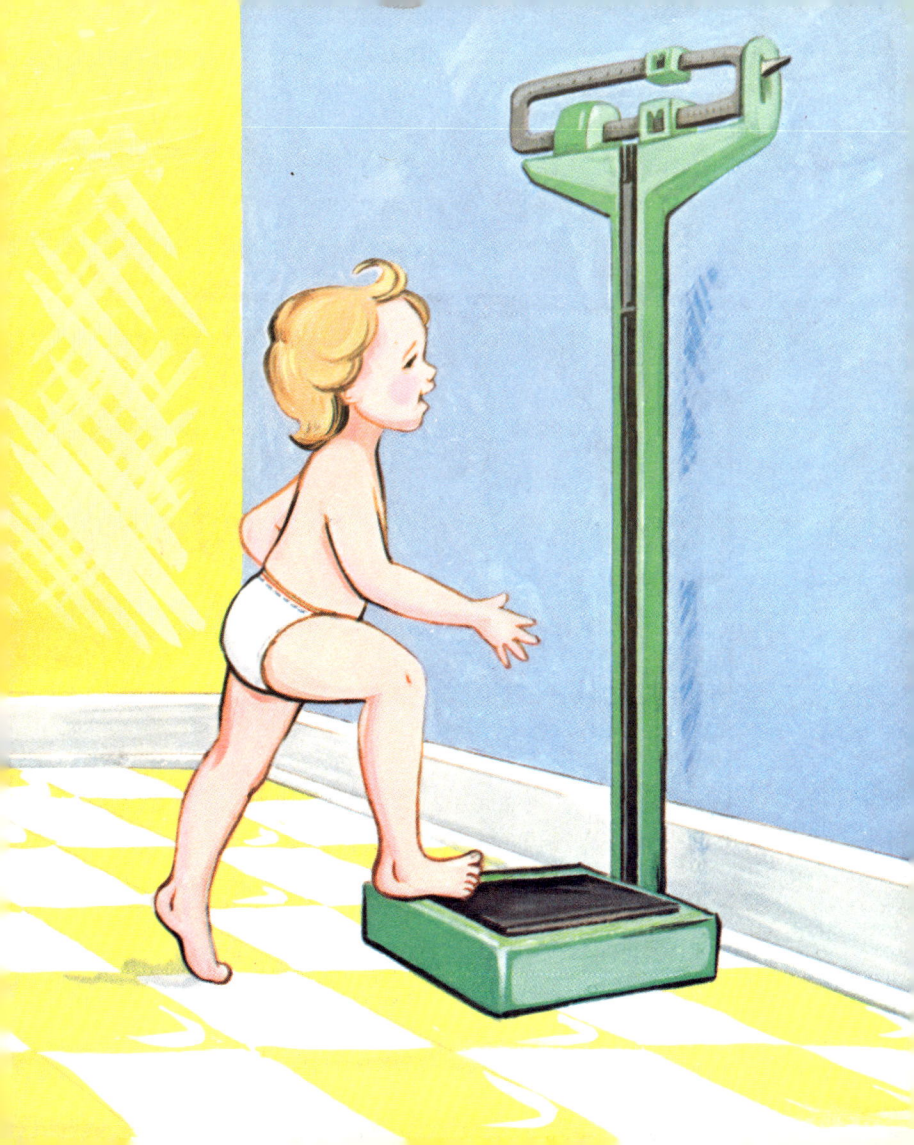

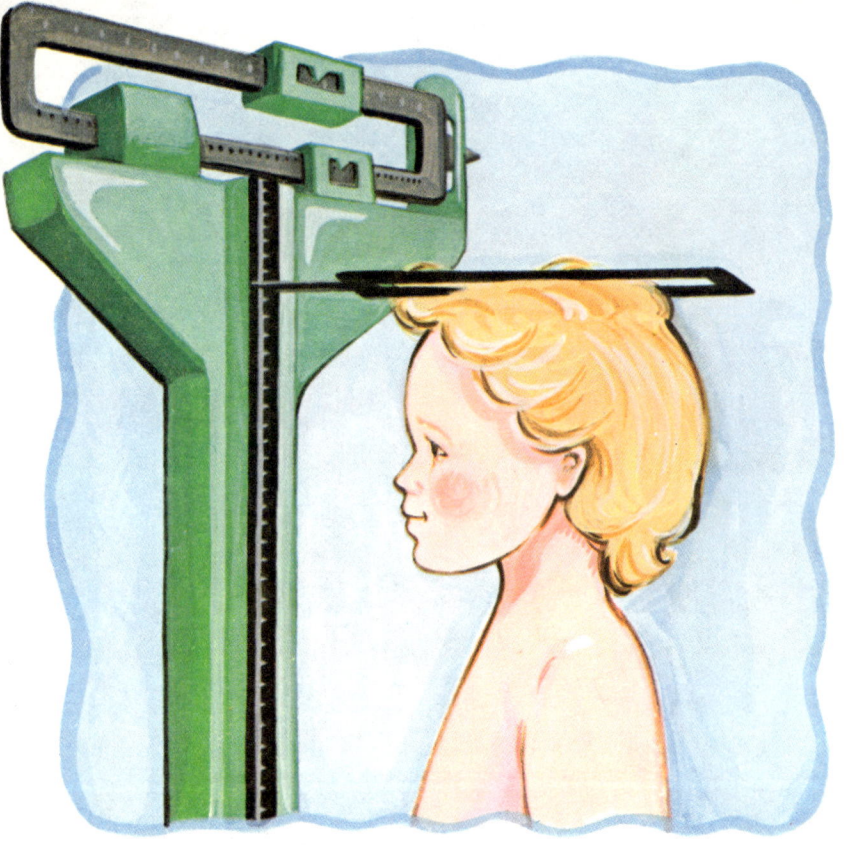

Dr. Smith moves the weights on the scale. Then she pulls out the measuring bar on the side of the scale and measures Simon.

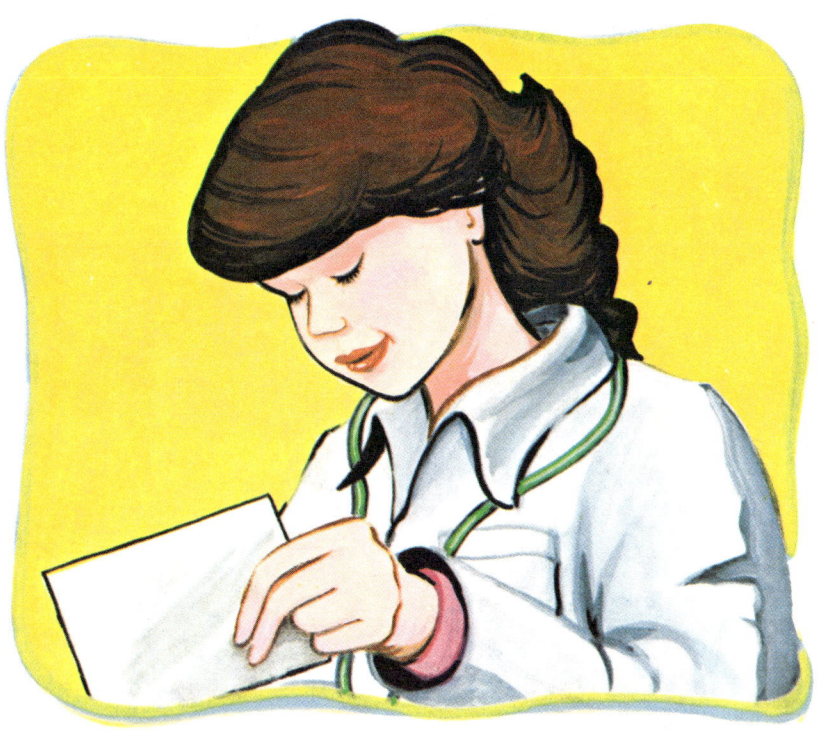

She looks at a white card. Simon's name is at the top.

"Good," Dr. Smith says. "You have gained four pounds and have grown one inch since your last checkup."

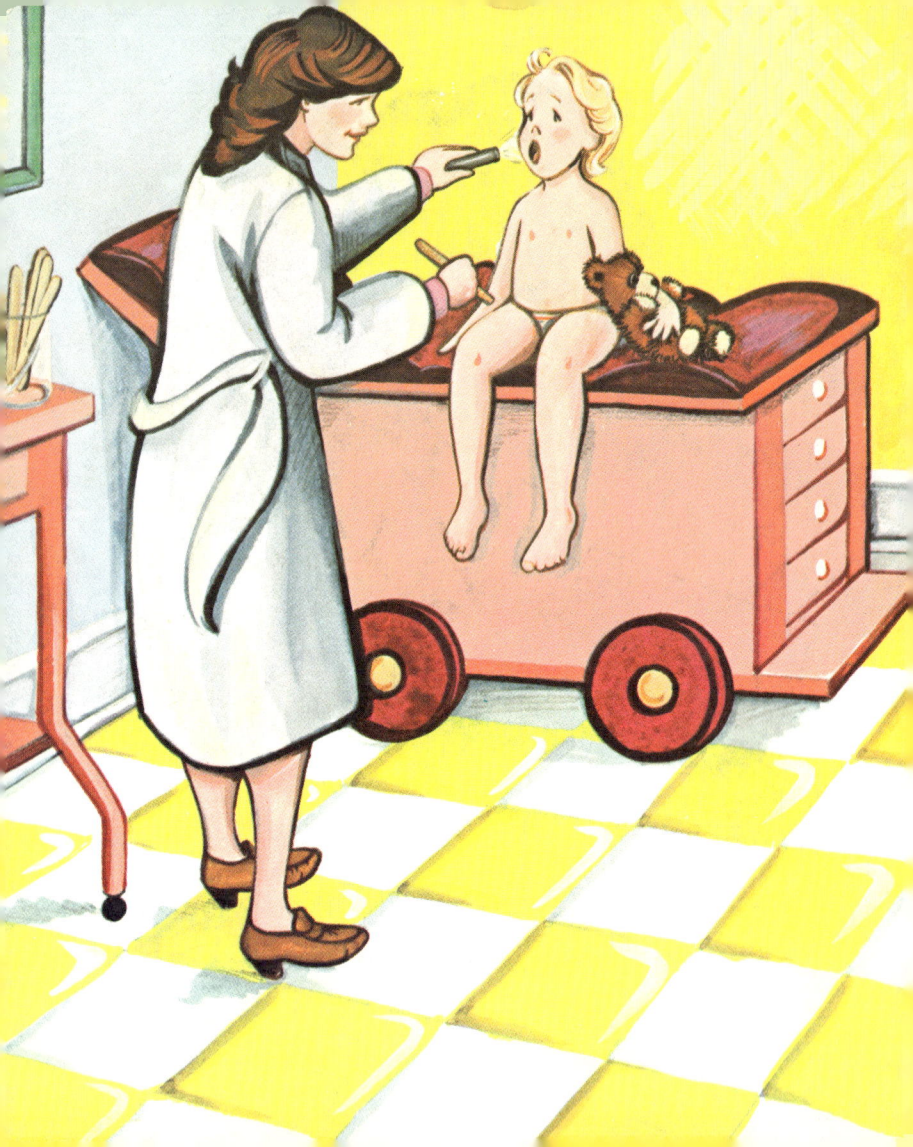

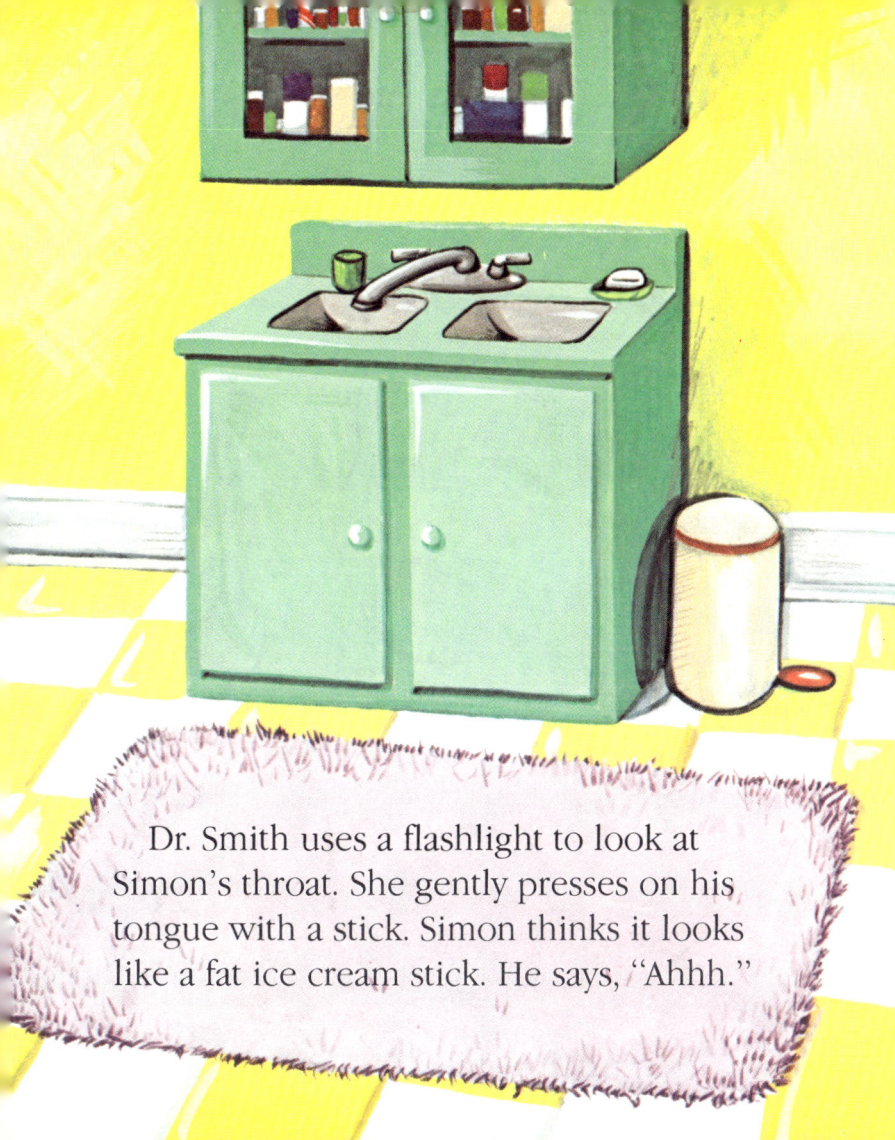

Dr. Smith uses a flashlight to look at Simon's throat. She gently presses on his tongue with a stick. Simon thinks it looks like a fat ice cream stick. He says, "Ahhh."

Then Dr. Smith looks into Simon's ears.

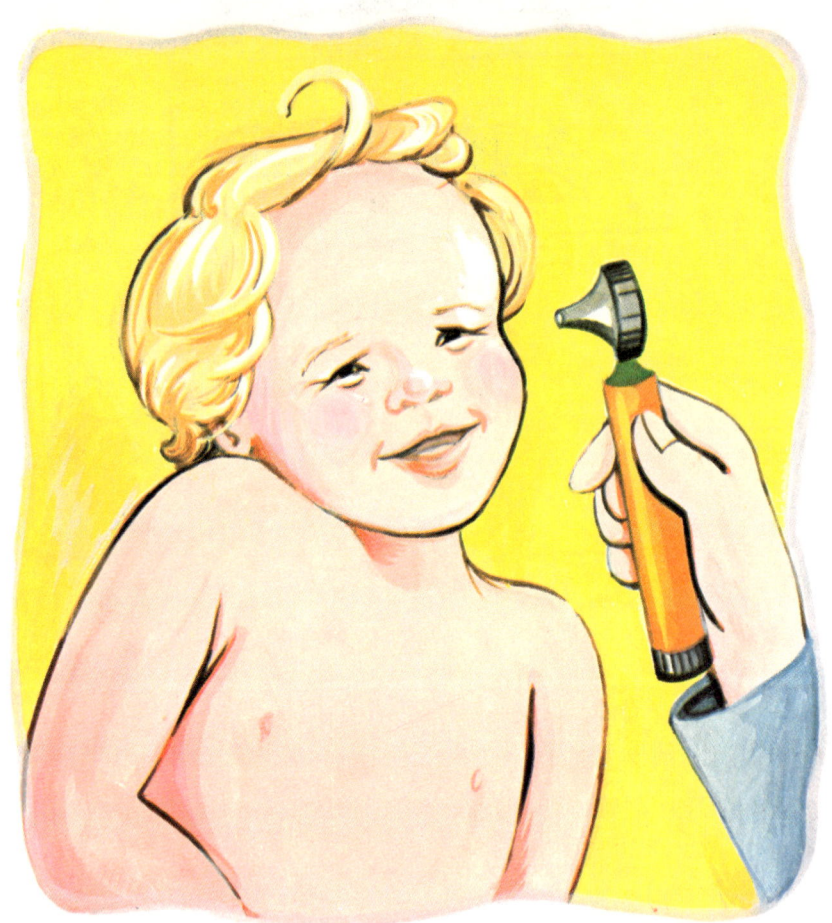

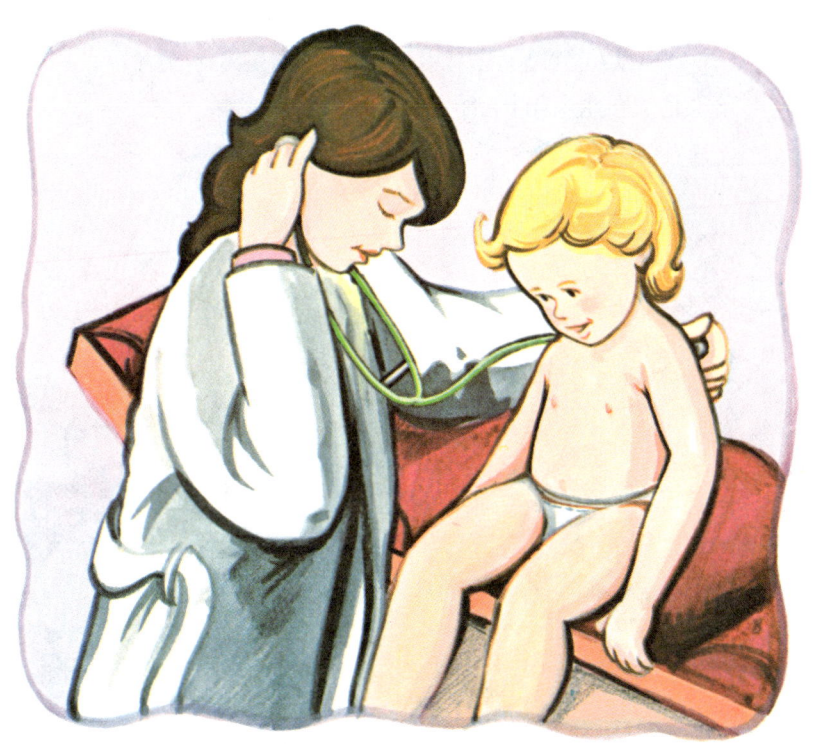

Dr. Smith asks Simon to cough and to take deep breaths. Dr. Smith listens to his chest and thumps his back with her fingers.

"You have a good, steady heartbeat and clear, healthy lungs," she tells Simon.

Next Dr. Smith feels Simon's tummy, his neck and under his arms.

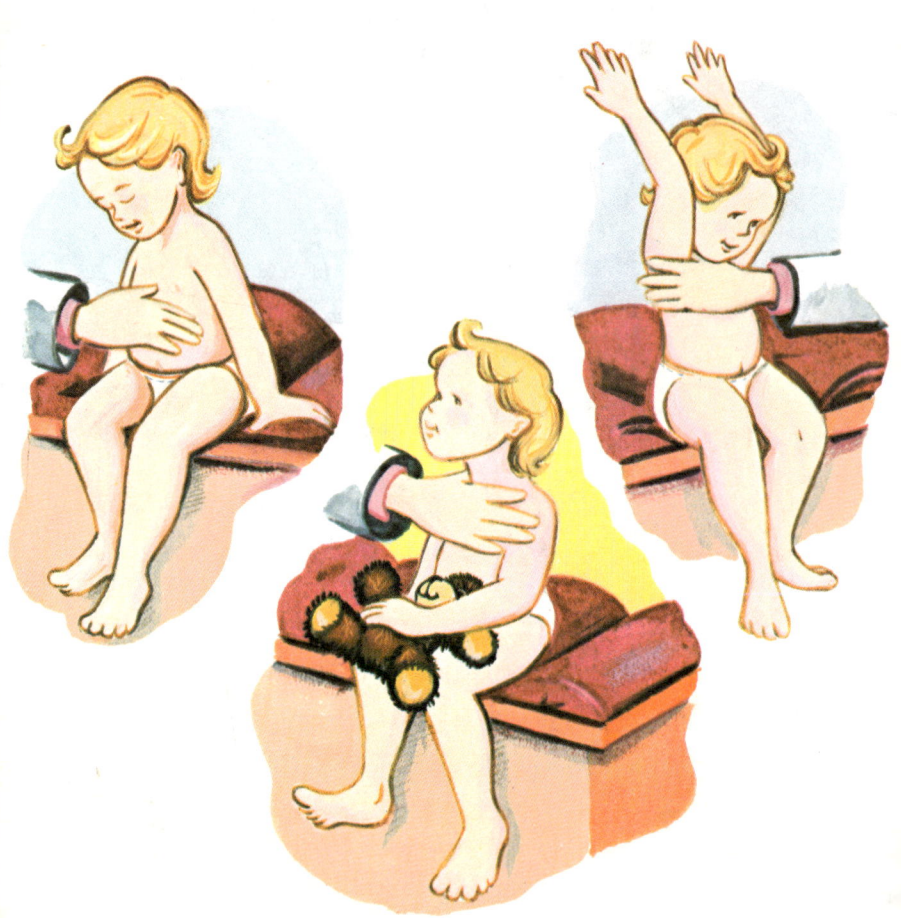

"You are growing well inside and out," she says.

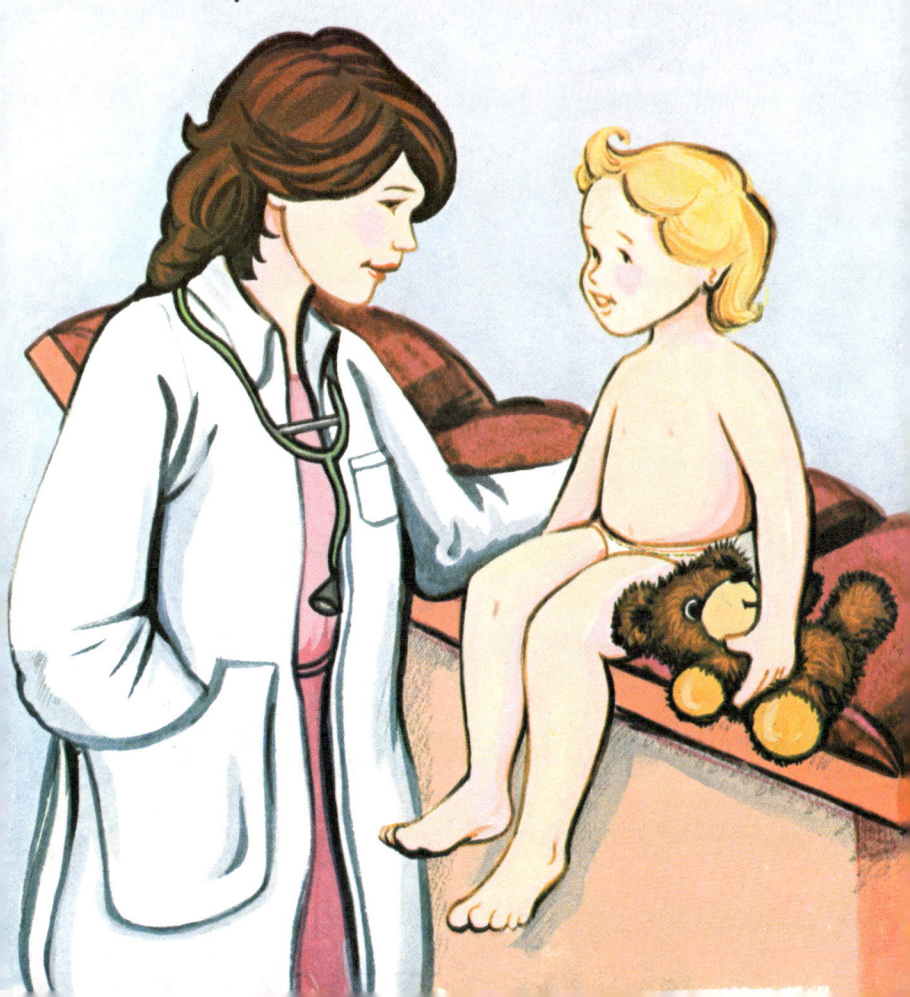

"Now it's time for your shot, Simon. You need a shot to keep you from getting some diseases. Cheer up! On your next visit, you won't need one."

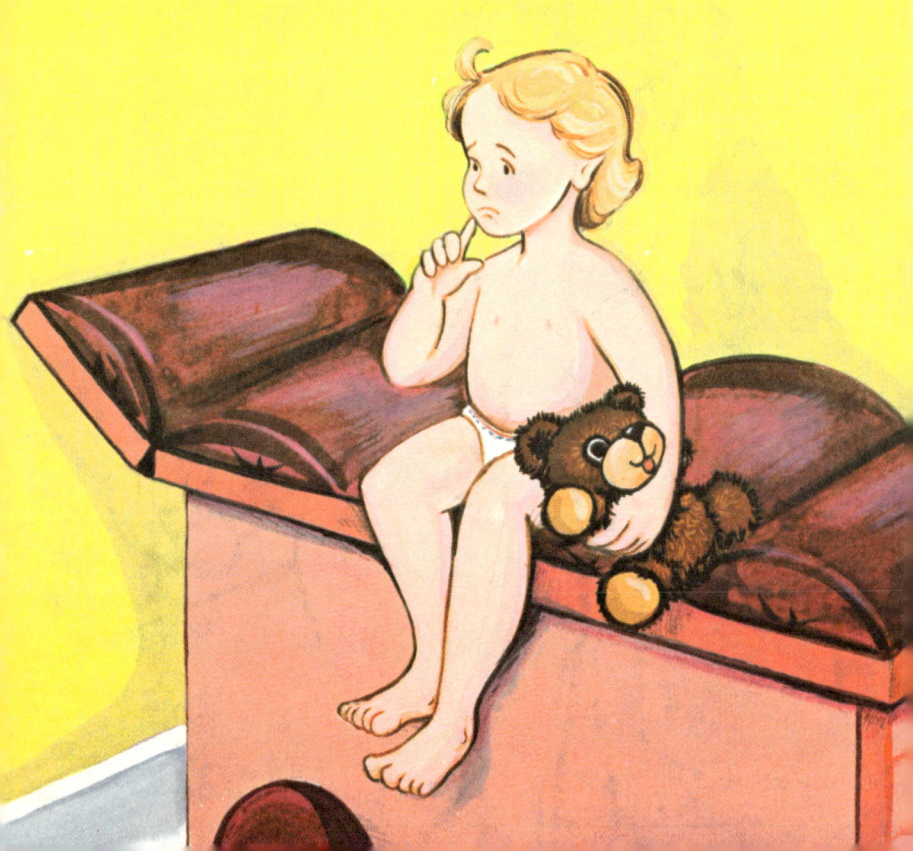

So Simon holds out his arm and closes his eyes tight.

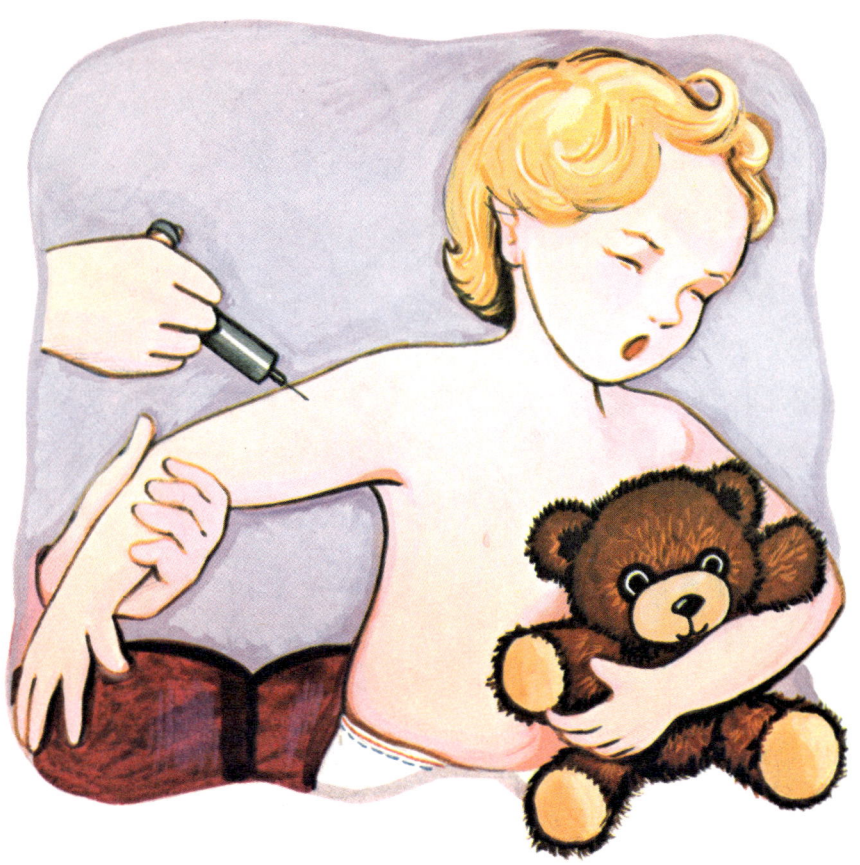

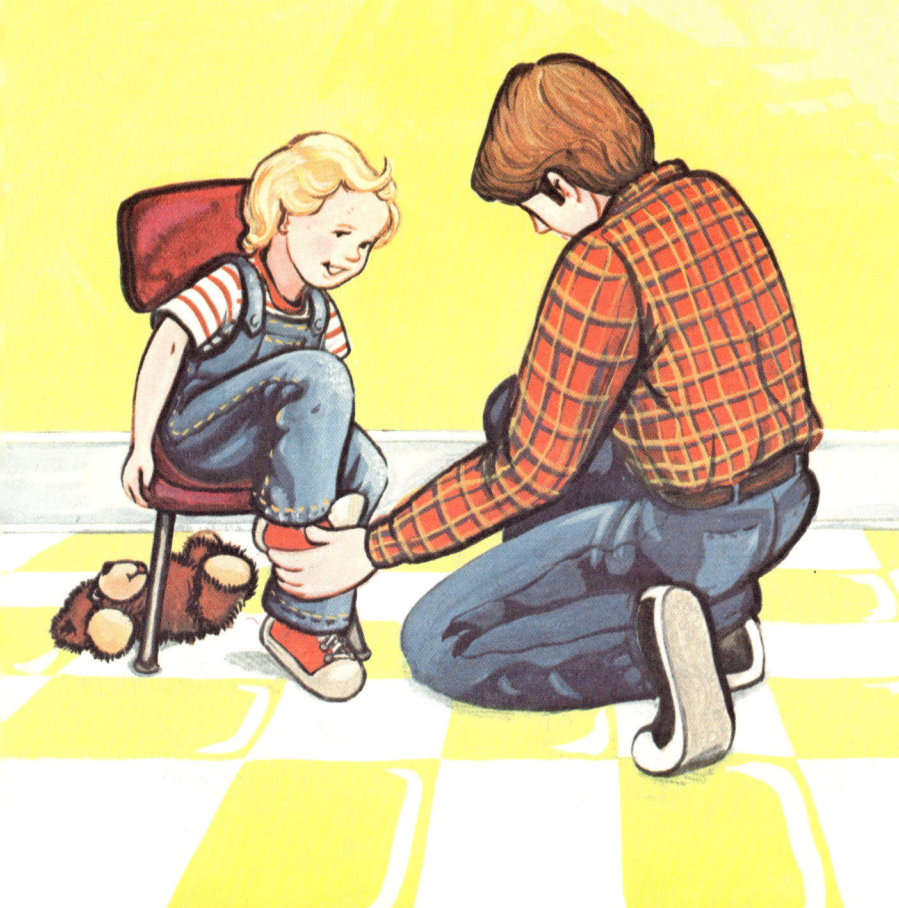

"We're all finished," says Dr. Smith.
Dad helps Simon get dressed.

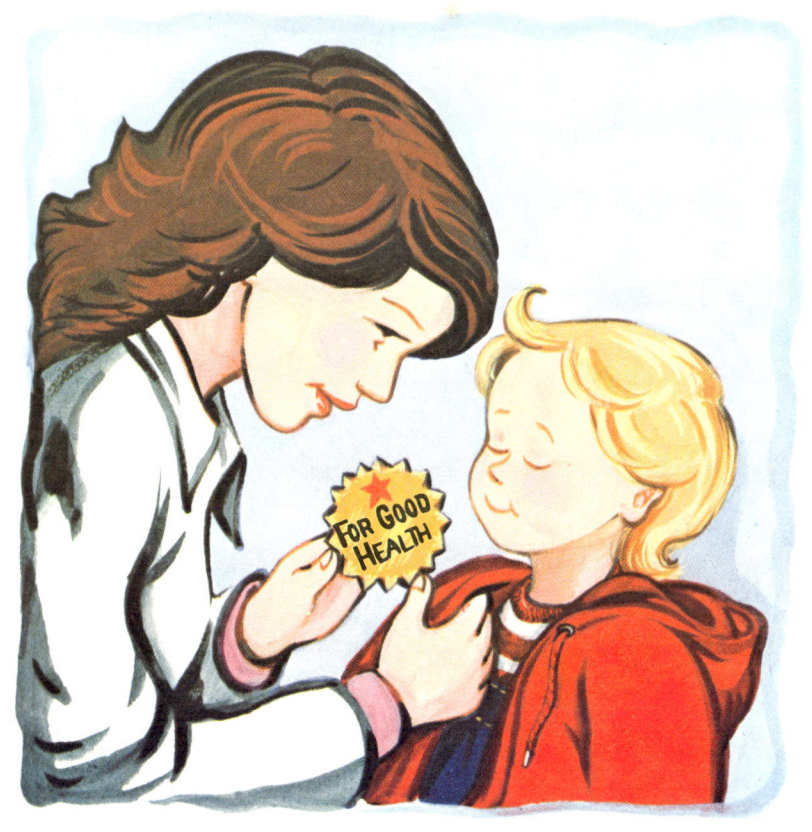

Dr. Smith says good-bye. She gives Simon a shiny sticker for his jacket.

In the waiting room Dad and Simon see a brand-new baby.
"Just wait," Simon whispers to the baby. "Soon you'll be big like me. Then you can get a sticker, too."

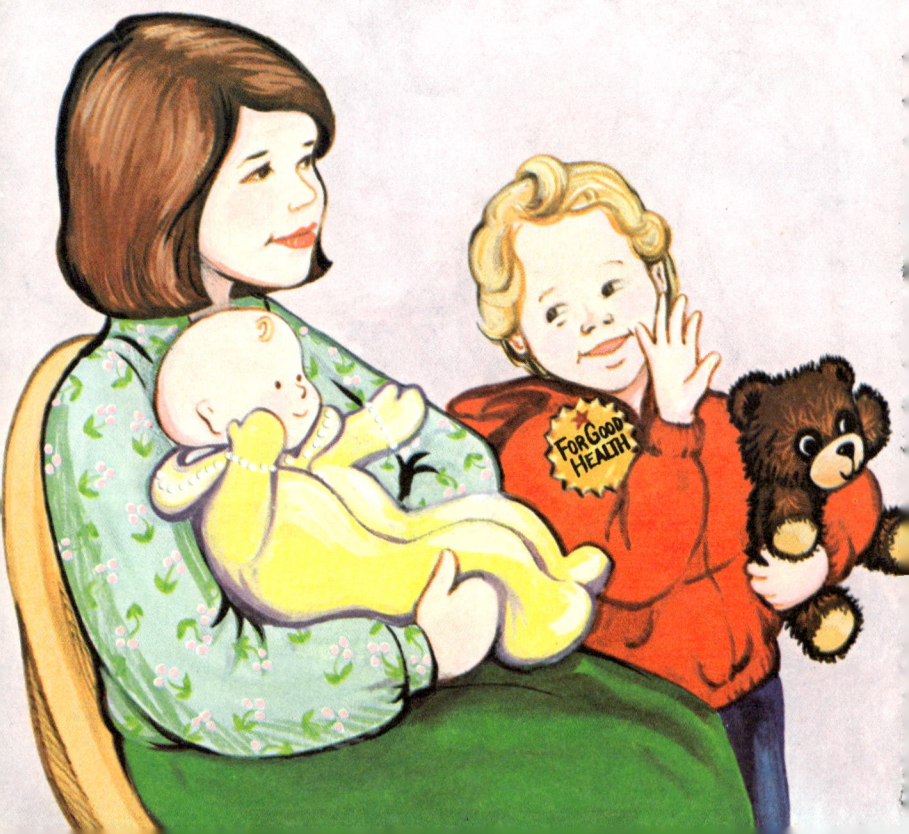